THE ALLERGIC PRINCESS

A Customizable Tale of Food Allergies

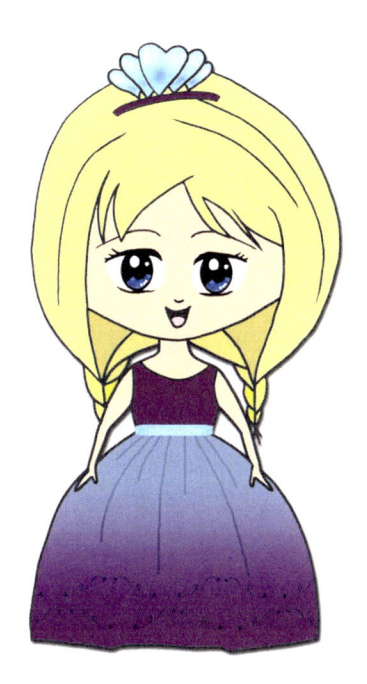

Written and Illustrated by

Jennifer Chung and Keira Chung

Copyright © 2016 by Jennifer Chung and Keira Chung. All rights reserved. No part of this book may be used or reproduced in any manner whatsoever without written permission except in the case of brief quotations in critical articles or reviews.

This is a work of fiction. Names, characters, businesses, places, events, and incidents are either the products of the author's imagination or used in a fictitious manner. Any resemblance to actual persons, living or dead, or actual events is purely coincidental.

This book is not intended as a substitute for the medical advice of physicians.

EpiPen® is a registered trademark of Mylan Inc. and Mylan Specialty L.P.
EpiPen® is an injection containing epinephrine that is used to treat severe allergic reactions.

www.AllergicPrincess.com

Available from Amazon.com and other online stores.

Summary: When Princess Isabella is tempted by multiple situations involving food, she learns to summon the willpower within to keep herself safe from allergic foods.

For:

Joe & Connor who believed in us

and

*The staff at Sean N. Parker Center for Allergy and Asthma Research
at Stanford University
for giving us the world.*

♥

How to customize this book:
To create a story to which your child can fully relate, use a ballpoint pen to fill in your child's allergic foods, symptoms, and safe snacks into the blank spaces on pages 14, 16, and 31.

This book belongs to:
_____

"Hooray! The day I've been waiting for is finally here!" yelled Princess Isabella as she climbed into the royal carriage.

Isabella's mommy had summoned the carriage to bring her to Princess Rose's birthday party.

5

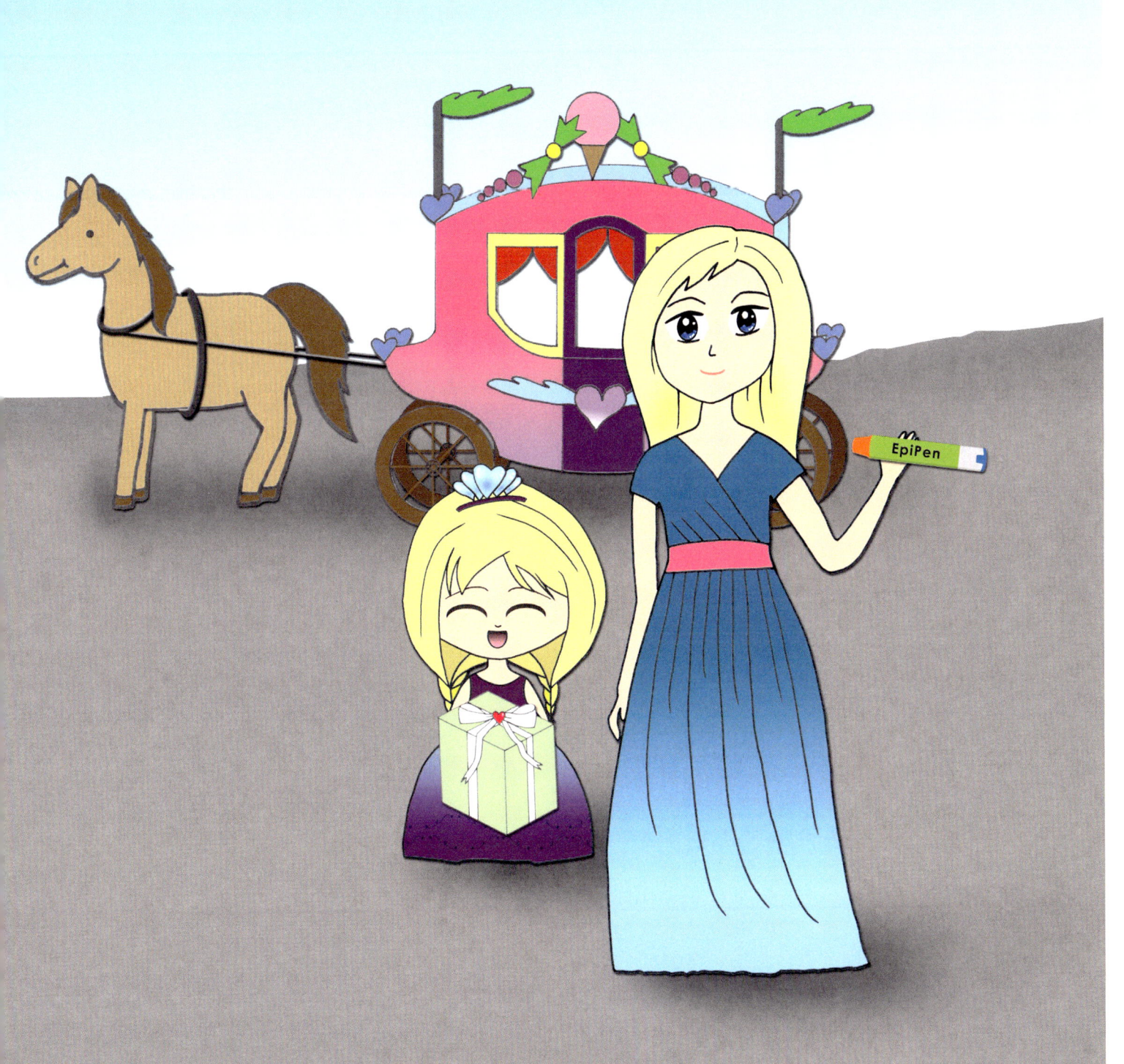

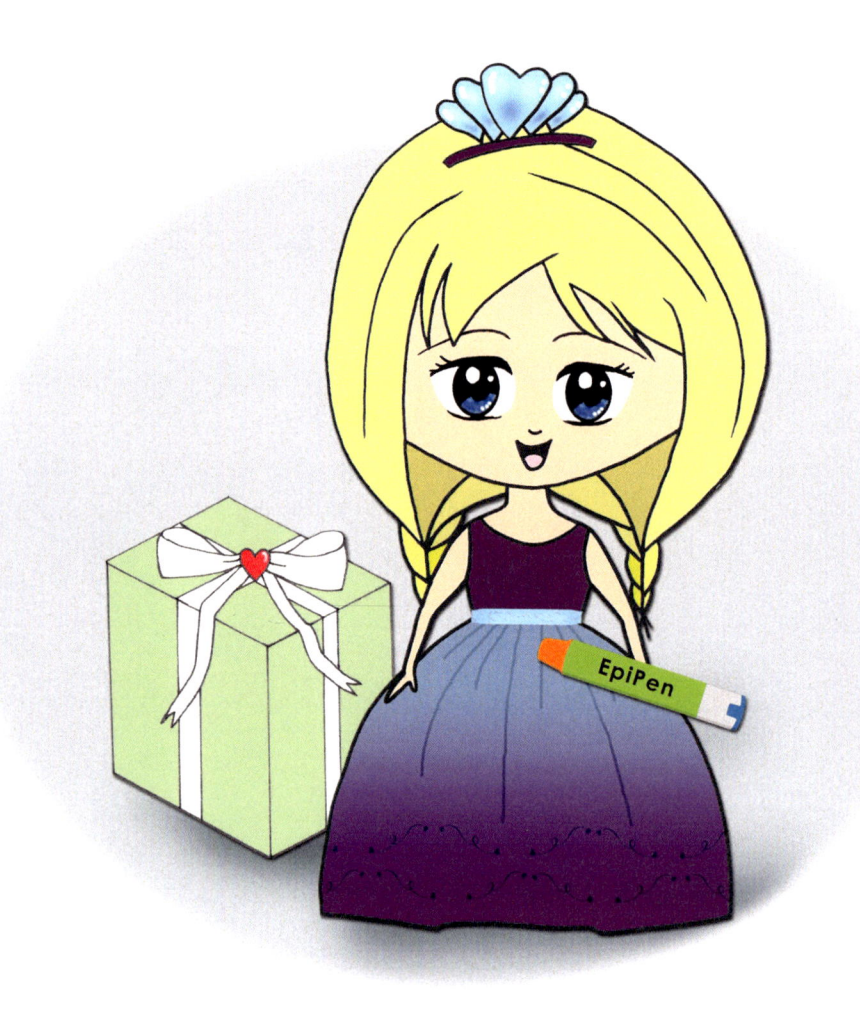

Along with a birthday present, Isabella also brought the EpiPen® that her doctor had given her for her food allergies. Her EpiPen® was her emergency medicine in case she accidentally ate food that she was allergic to.

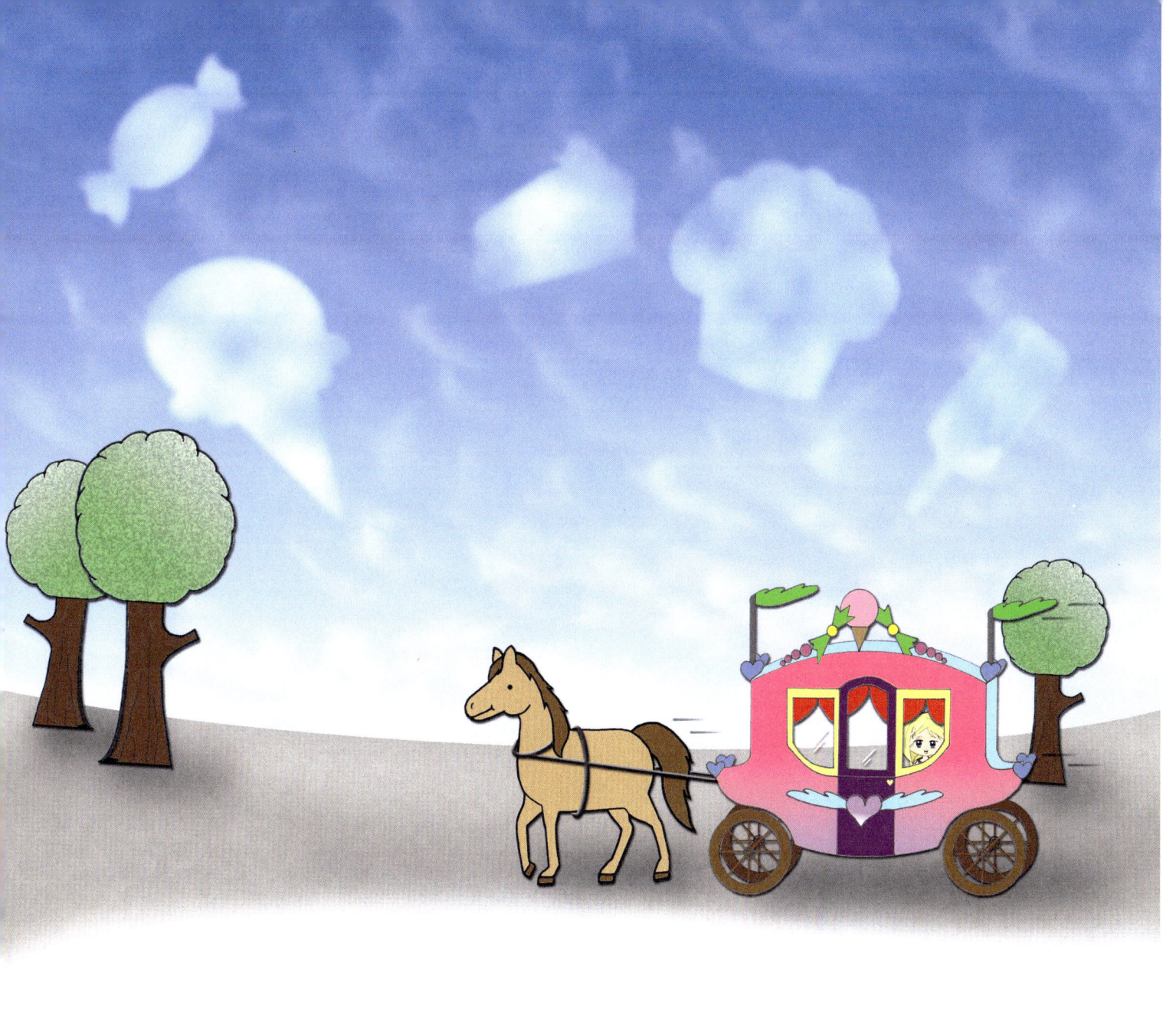

Looking out the window of the carriage,
Isabella watched as cloud shapes passed by.

It felt like the longest ride ever, until Isabella finally spotted Rose's castle. As she passed through the castle gate, her heart raced faster. What will the party be like? She wondered. Will I be allergic to the cake?

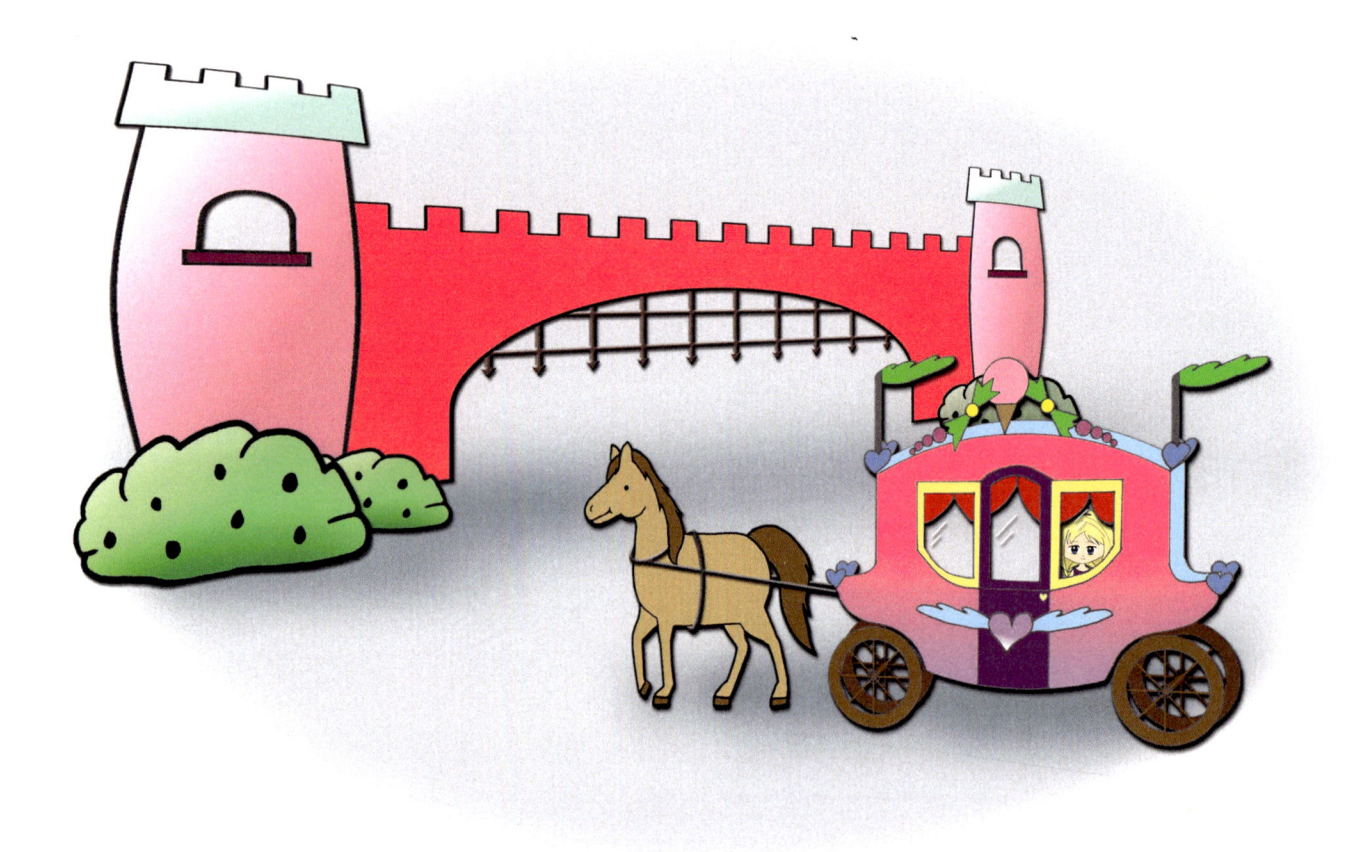

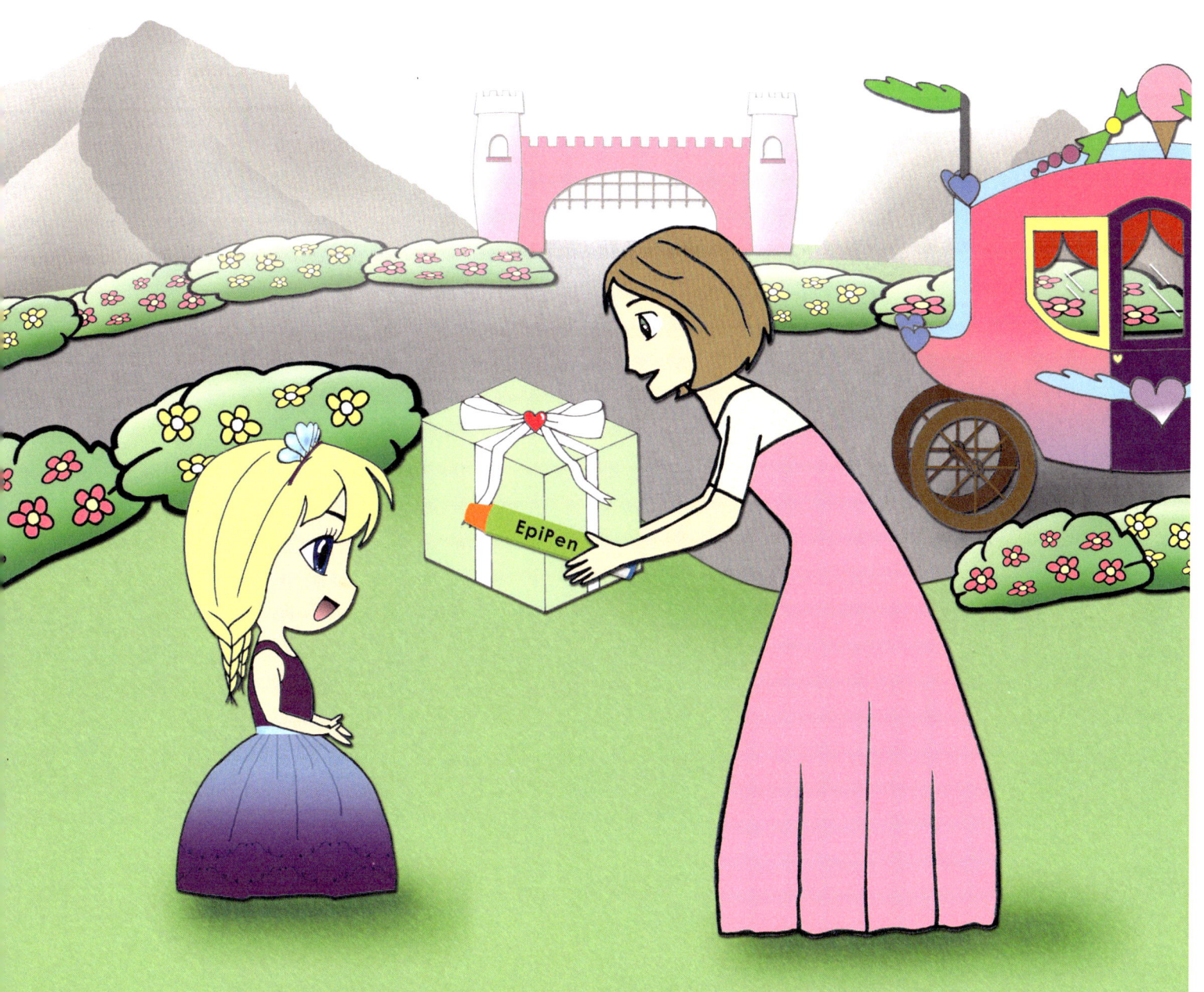

At last, the carriage came to a stop and Isabella excitedly hopped off. She handed both the EpiPen® and the birthday present to Rose's mommy, who came to welcome her into their castle grounds.

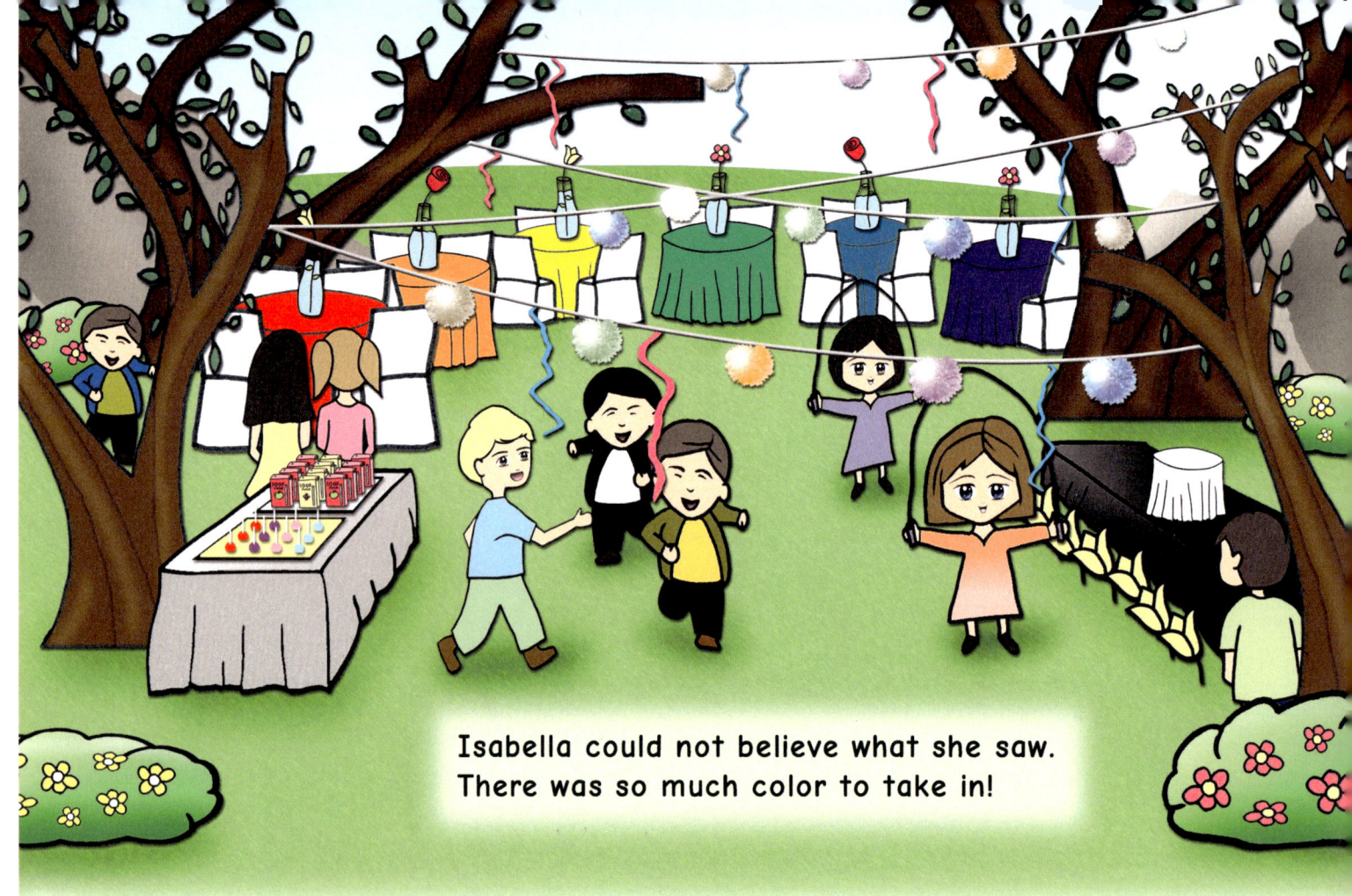

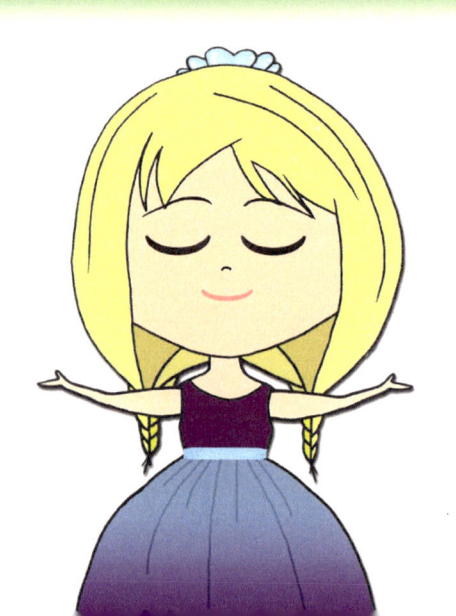

Isabella could not believe what she saw. There was so much color to take in!

To savor the moment, she closed her eyes and took a deep breath. Children's laughter and the smell of flowers surrounded her.

Rose waved and called out, "Isabella! Over here!"

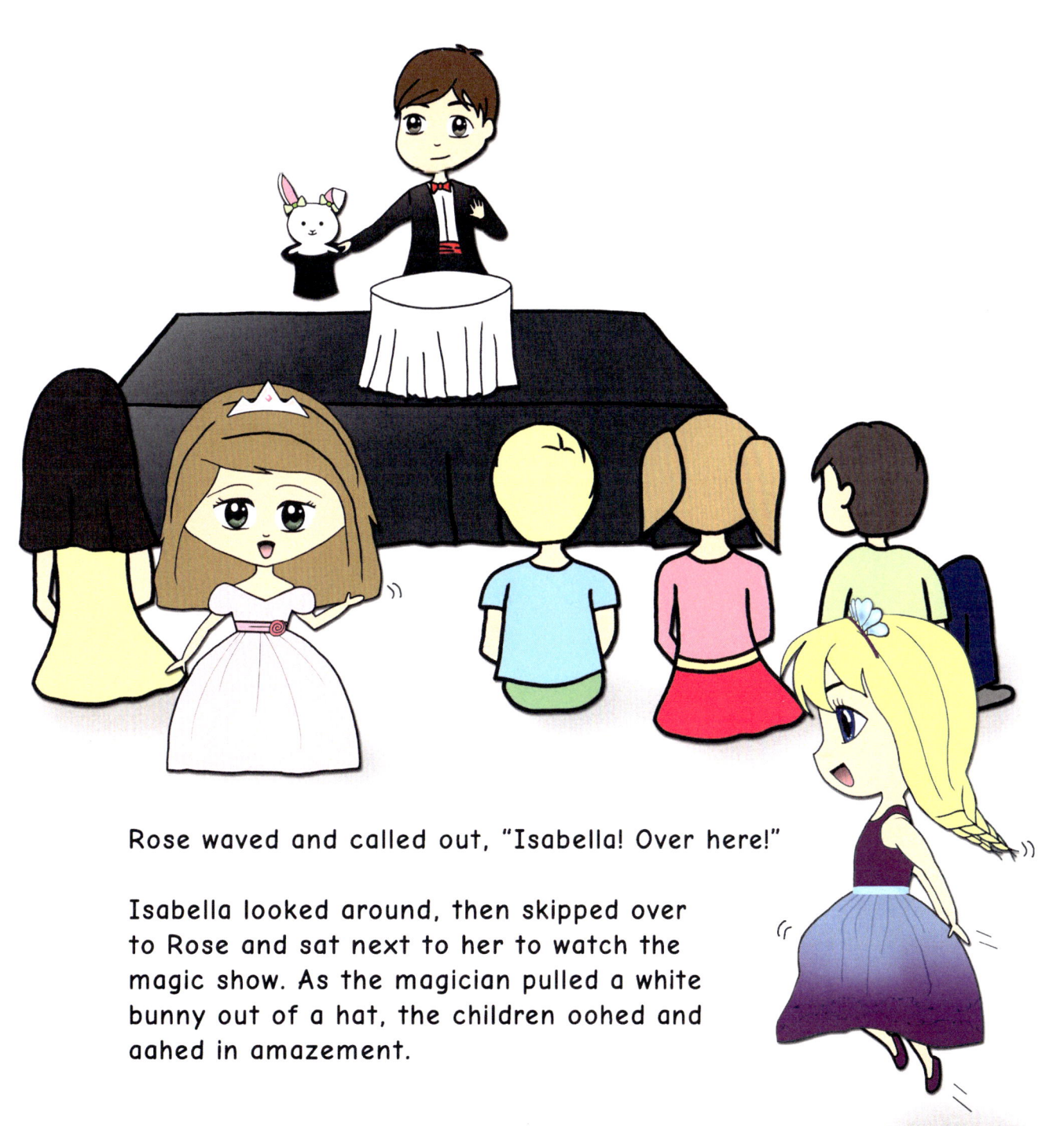

Isabella looked around, then skipped over to Rose and sat next to her to watch the magic show. As the magician pulled a white bunny out of a hat, the children oohed and aahed in amazement.

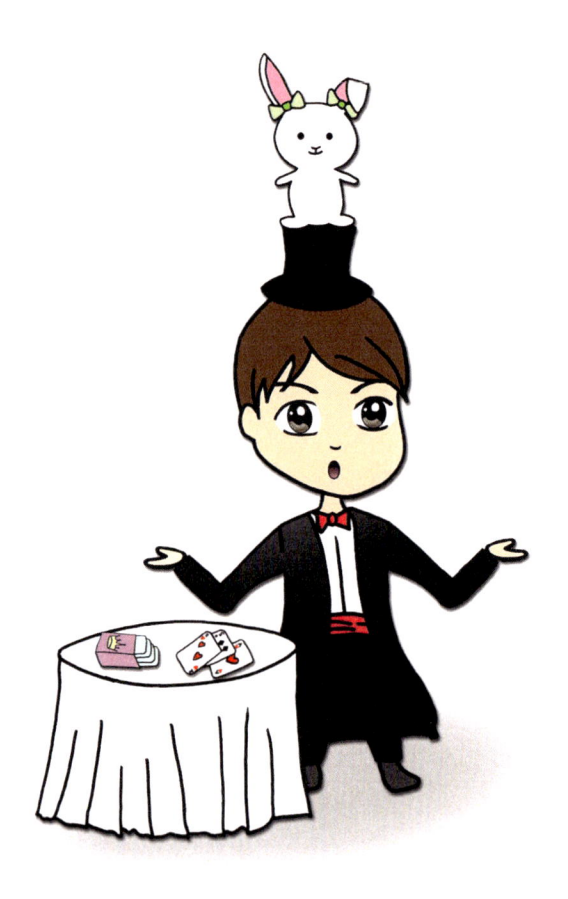

To prepare for his next trick, the magician placed the bunny on the table and went to find his deck of cards. Without warning, the bunny hopped away.

The magician looked around and asked the children, "Do you know where my bunny went?"

All at once, the children started laughing.

After the fun-filled magic show, it was time for the birthday cake. Isabella squealed as she jumped up and down, clapping her hands. Three magnificent layers of pink cake decorated with frosting flowers and pearl sprinkles stood before her.

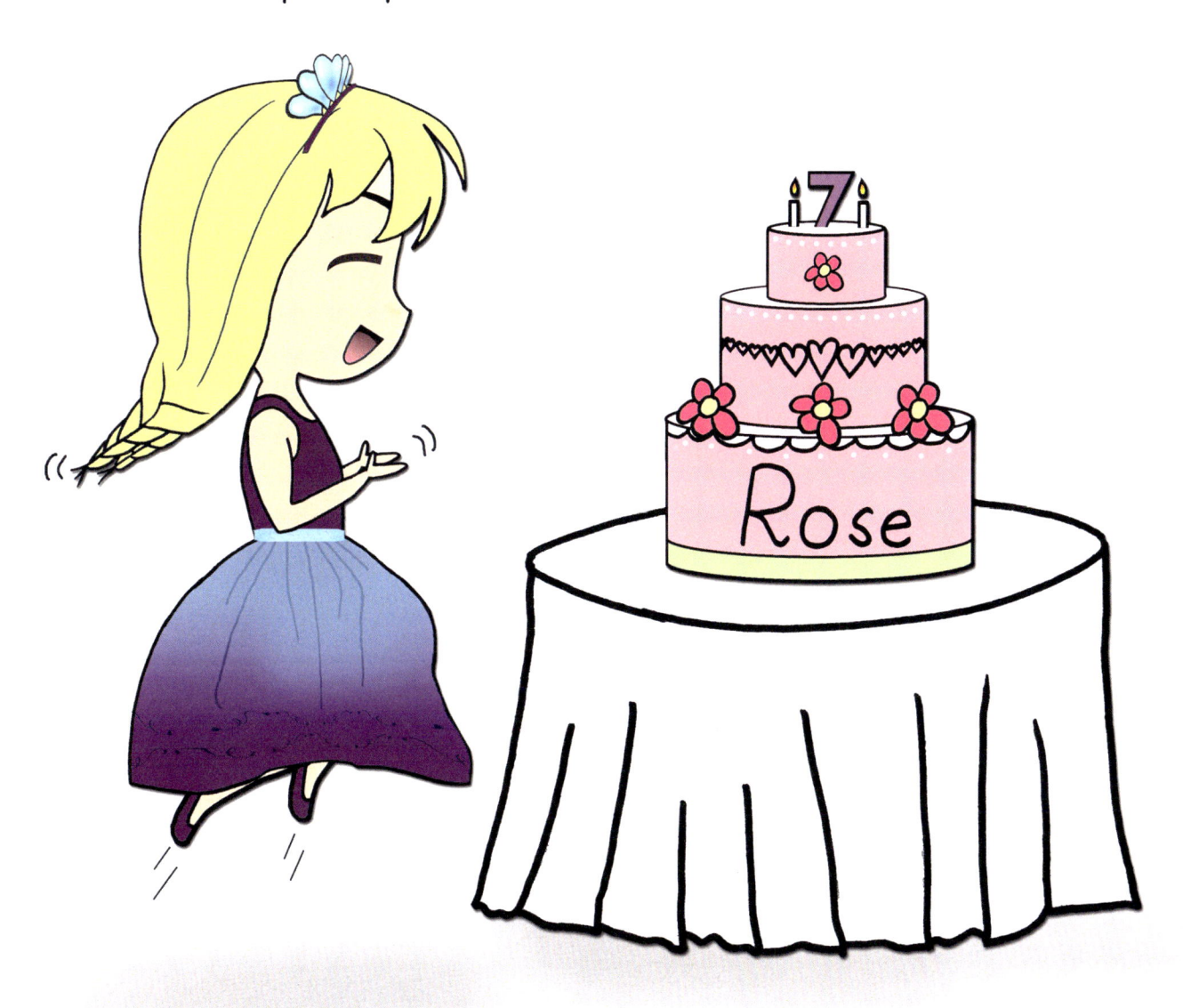

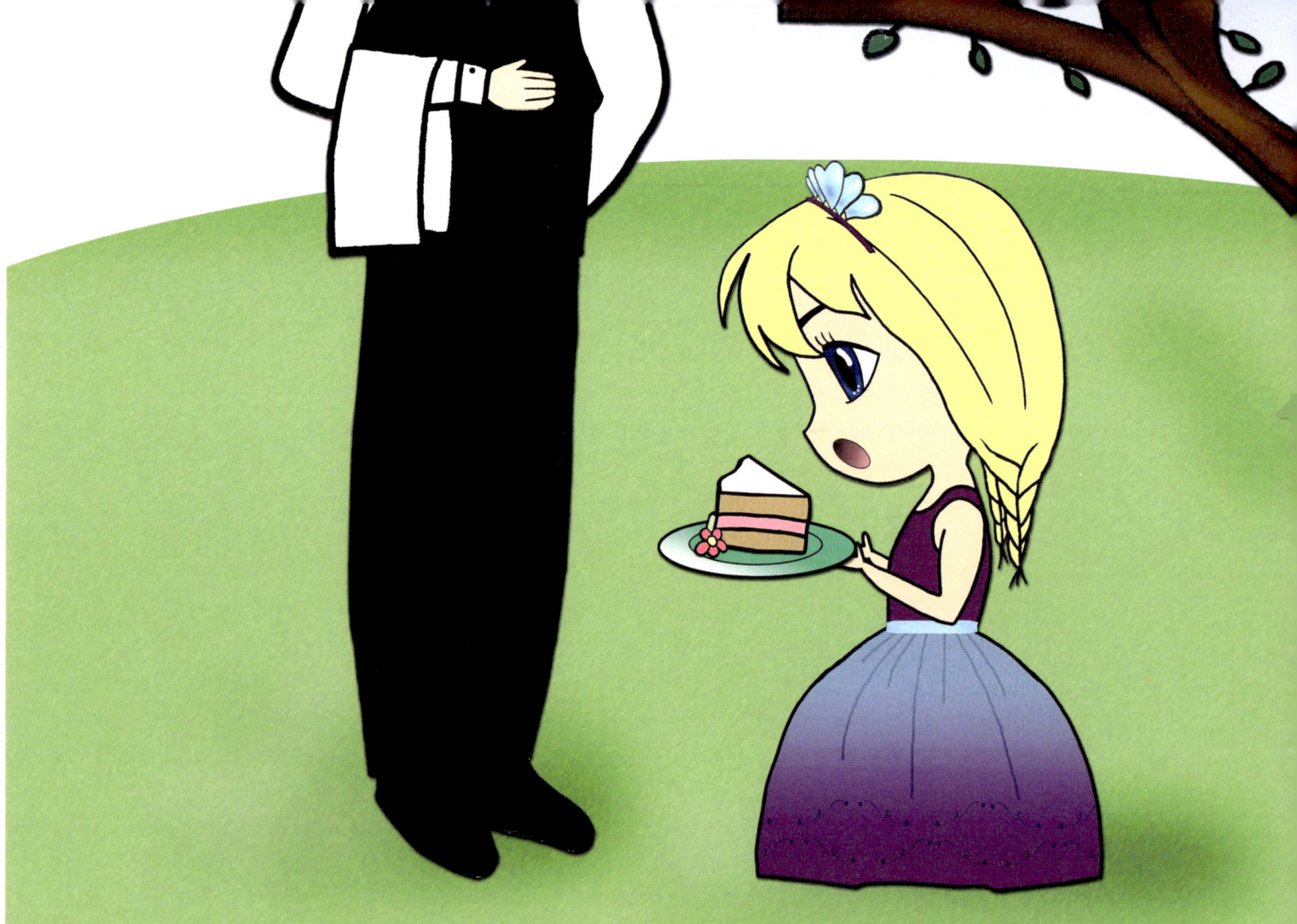

Isabella stared with huge eyes at the piece of cake that was handed to her. What should I do? What *can* I do? She remembered her food allergies, but the cake looked both delicious and so harmless.

She did not see any _____
in the cake.   [fill in allergic foods here]

Standing alone, Isabella glanced around as she held the slice of cake. She took a chance and scooped the biggest bite ever and placed it in her mouth. It was scrumptious!

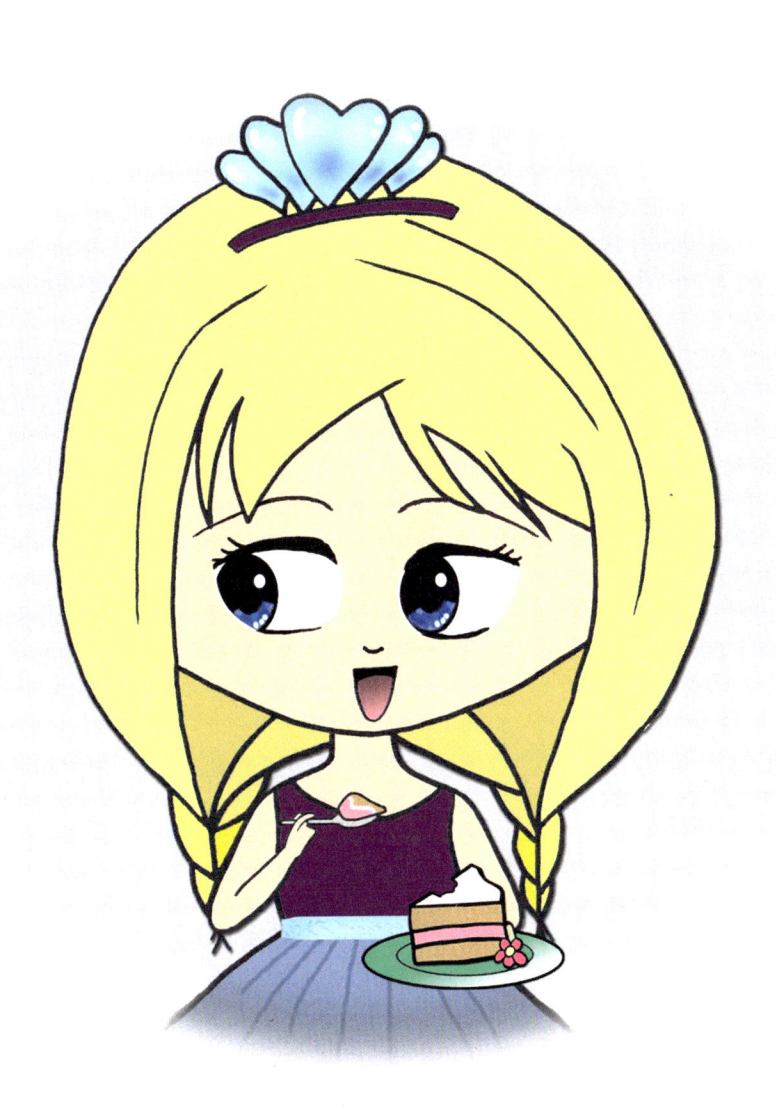

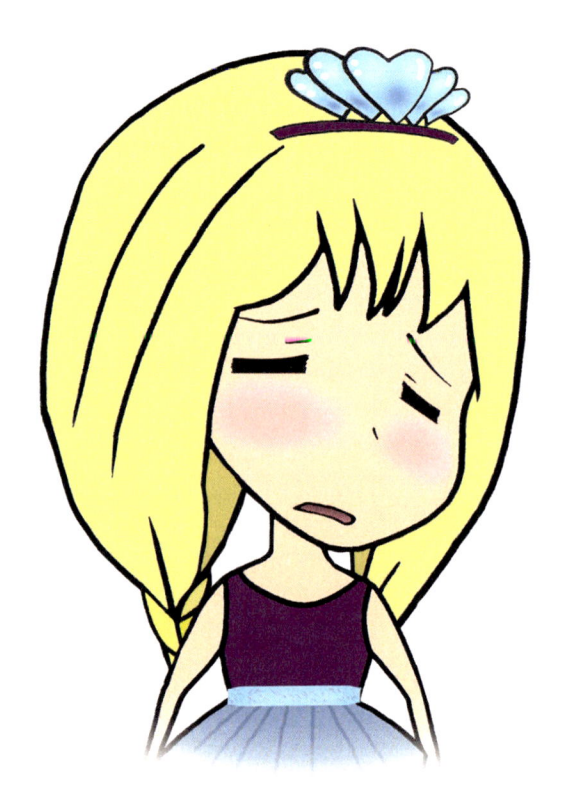

In an instant, everything changed. Isabella felt sick and realized that she was having an allergic reaction.

She recognized the symptoms of _____.
She needed help!
[fill in allergic symptoms here]

Isabella ran to the butler and told him, "I'm having an allergic reaction... and I need my EpiPen®!"

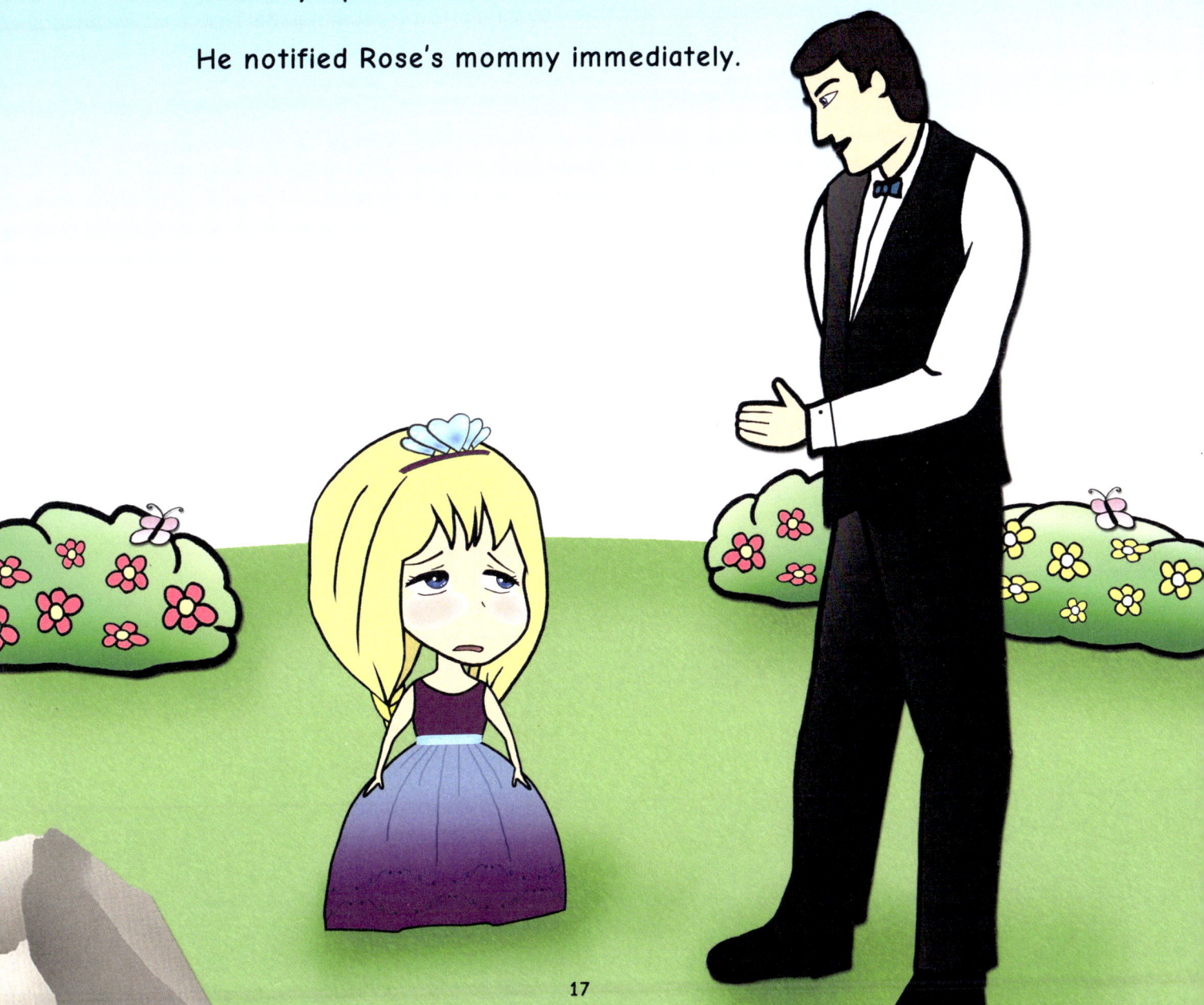

He notified Rose's mommy immediately.

Rose's mommy rushed over and injected the EpiPen® into Isabella's leg.

Rose came over to see what all the commotion was about and saw that her friend was in trouble. She wanted to stay with Isabella, but realized she had to do a very important job first.

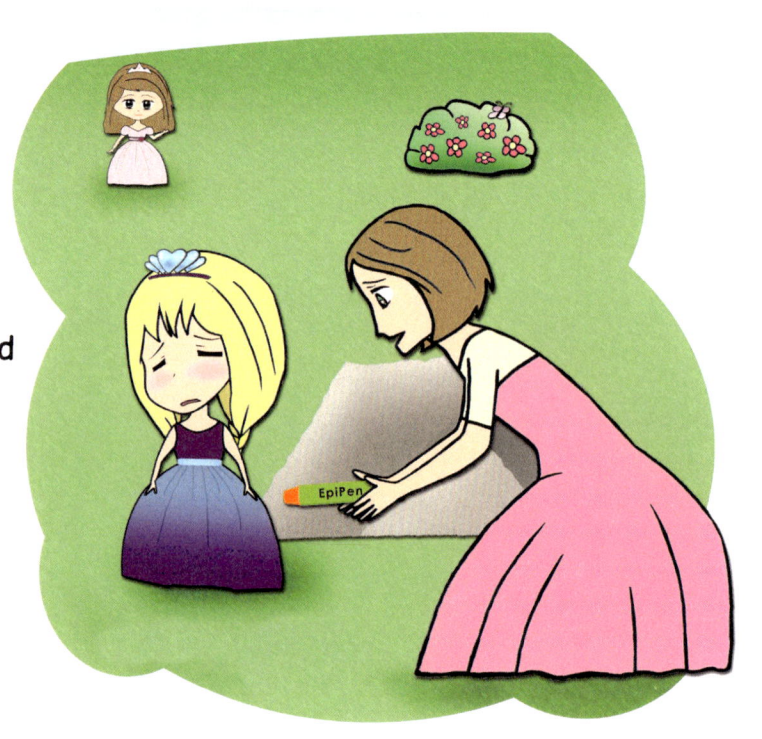

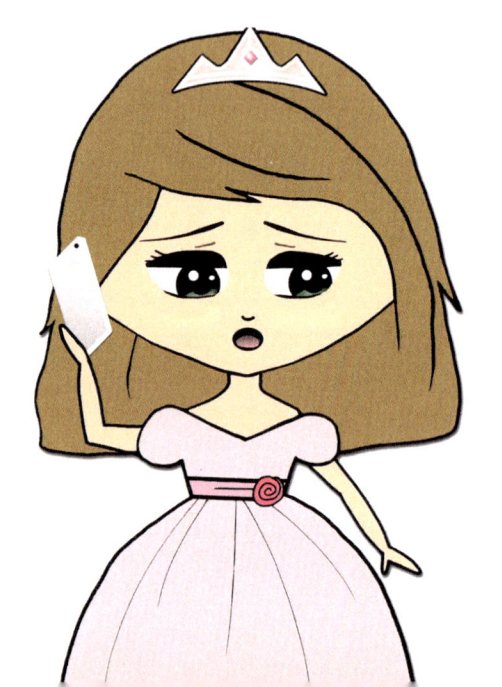

She went to the phone and called Isabella's mommy to tell her what had happened.

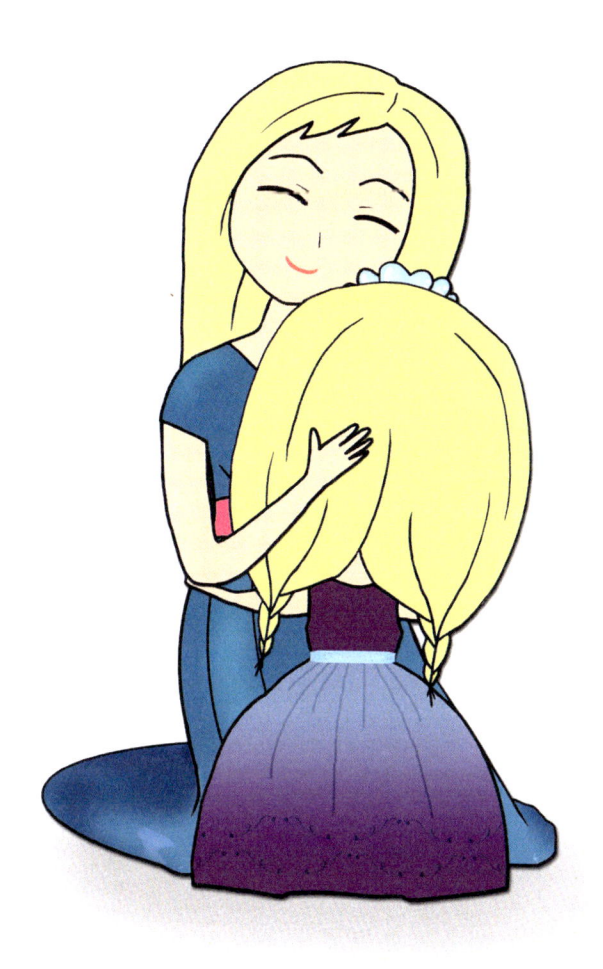

Although she was still scared, Isabella began to feel better. When her mommy finally arrived to bring her to the Royal Hospital, Isabella sank into her arms.

"I'm so glad you're here," whispered Isabella.

That night, after the hospital visit, Isabella was glad to go home so that she could cuddle with her favorite teddy bear. She ate a quick dinner and went to bed early to have a good night of sleep.

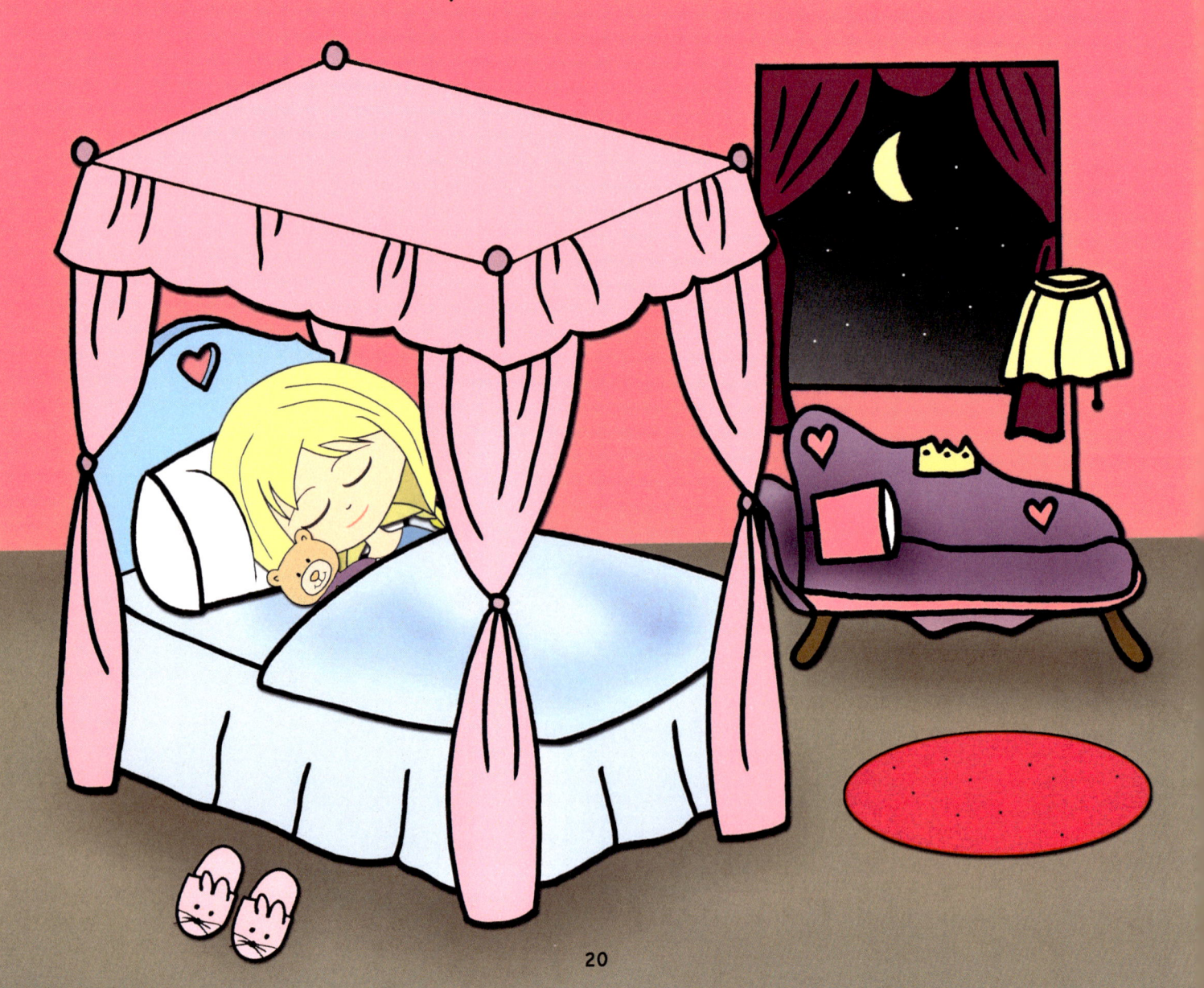

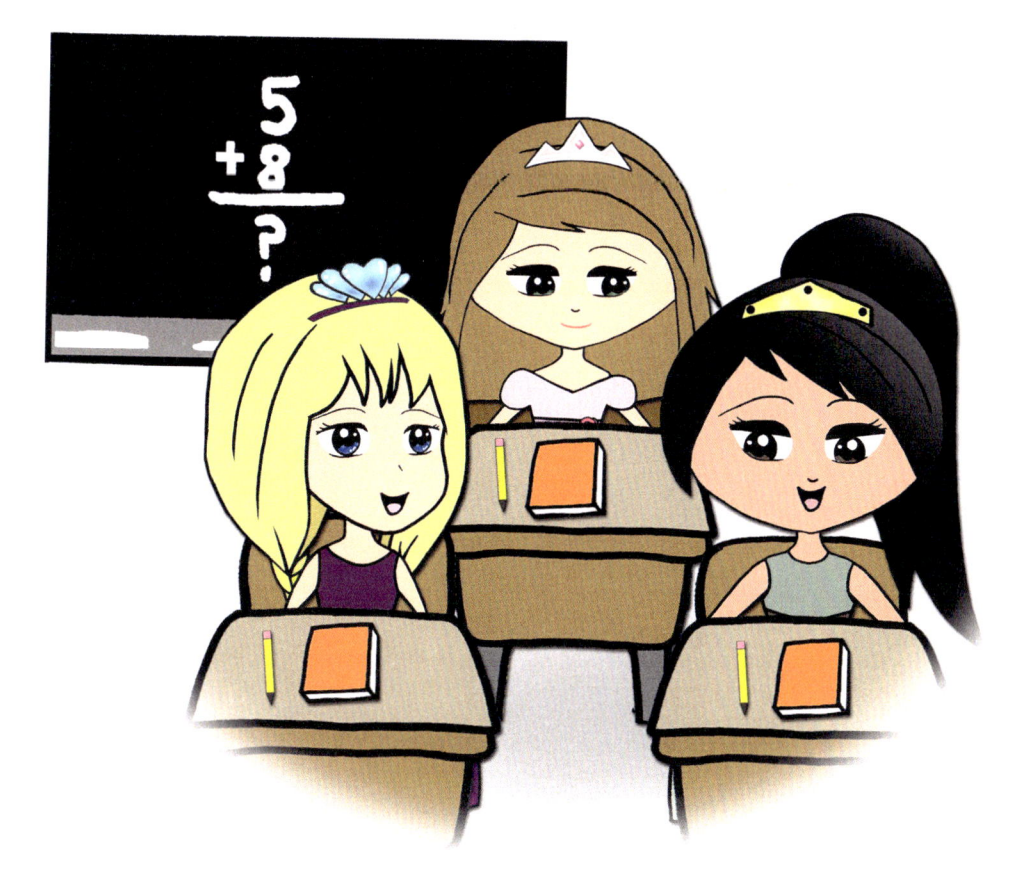

The next morning, Isabella woke up feeling refreshed. She got dressed and ate breakfast, then hopped onto the carriage, ready for a new day at school. When she reached Royal Academy School, she noticed a new girl she had never seen before. Her name was Princess Lexi.

"Lexi, want to come to my castle for a play date tomorrow?" asked Isabella. "Rose will be there too."

"That would be lovely, I will ask my mother," replied Lexi.

When Lexi and her mommy arrived at Isabella's castle, Isabella and Rose were already playing hopscotch. They quickly ran over to greet Lexi.

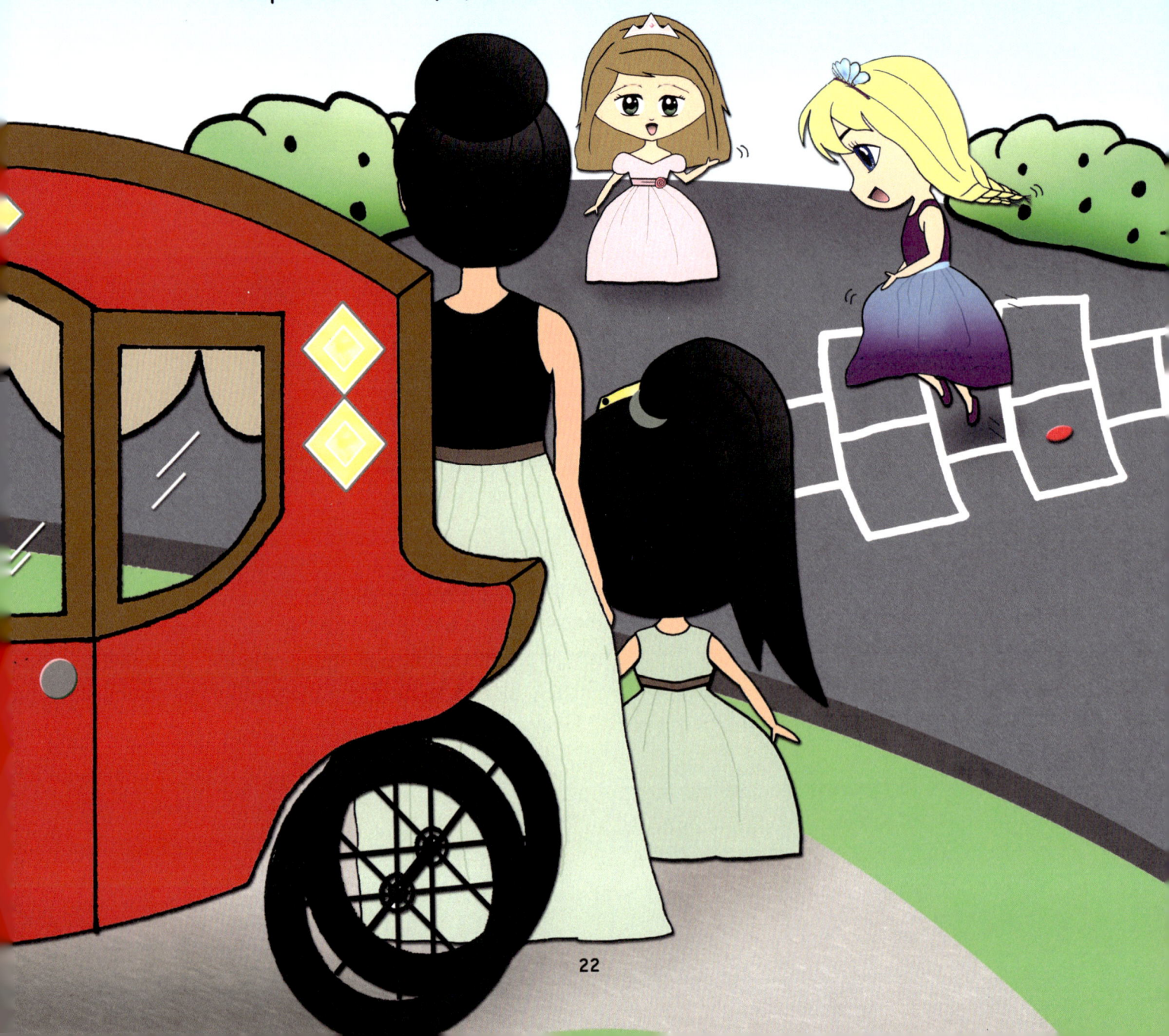

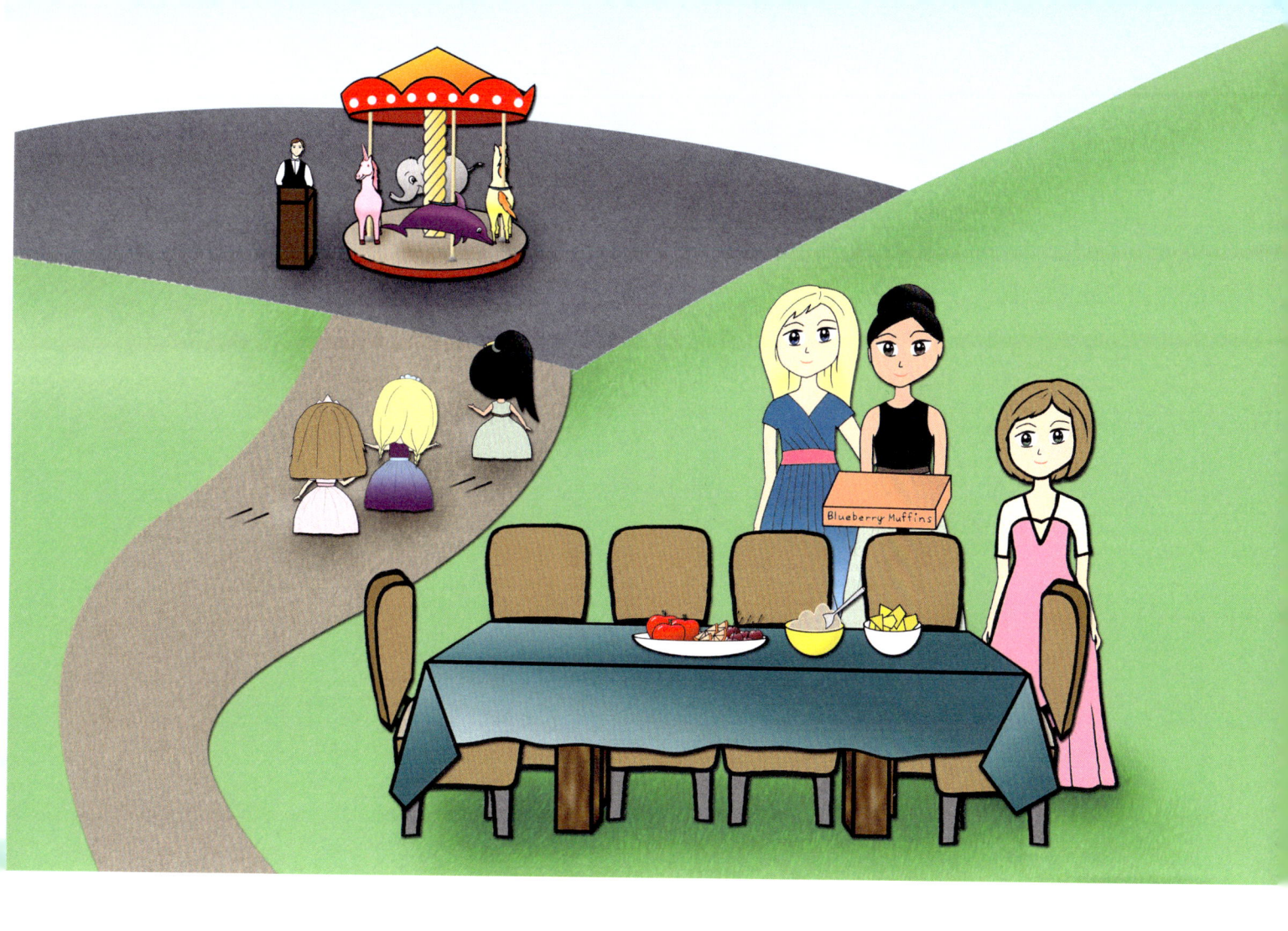

The three girls raced to the carousel while the three mommies sat down for a nice long chat.

"I would like the yellow horse," stated Lexi.

"Purple dolphin, you're mine!" cried Isabella.

"The pink unicorn for me!" shouted Rose.

23

The music began and off the girls went! The carousel spun faster and faster, around and around, again and again.

"Woohoo! This is the best!" cried Rose.

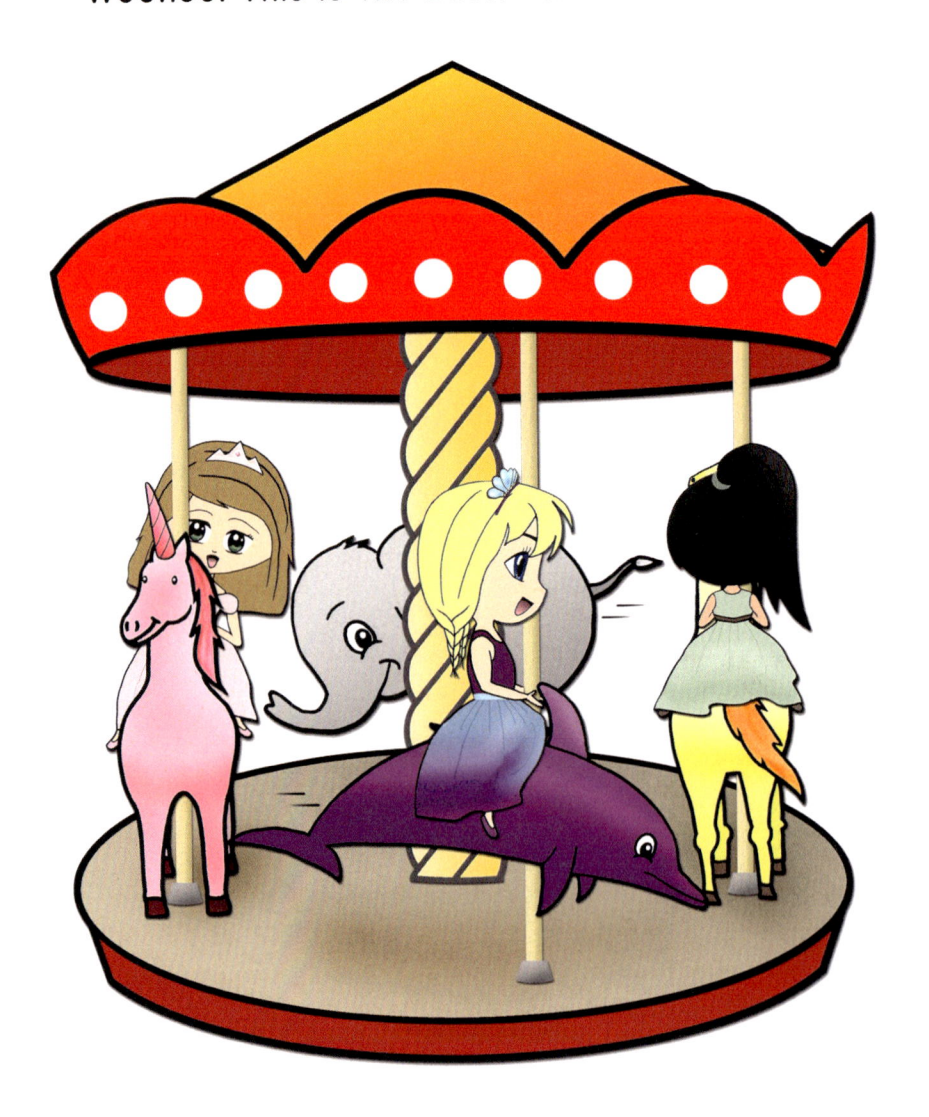

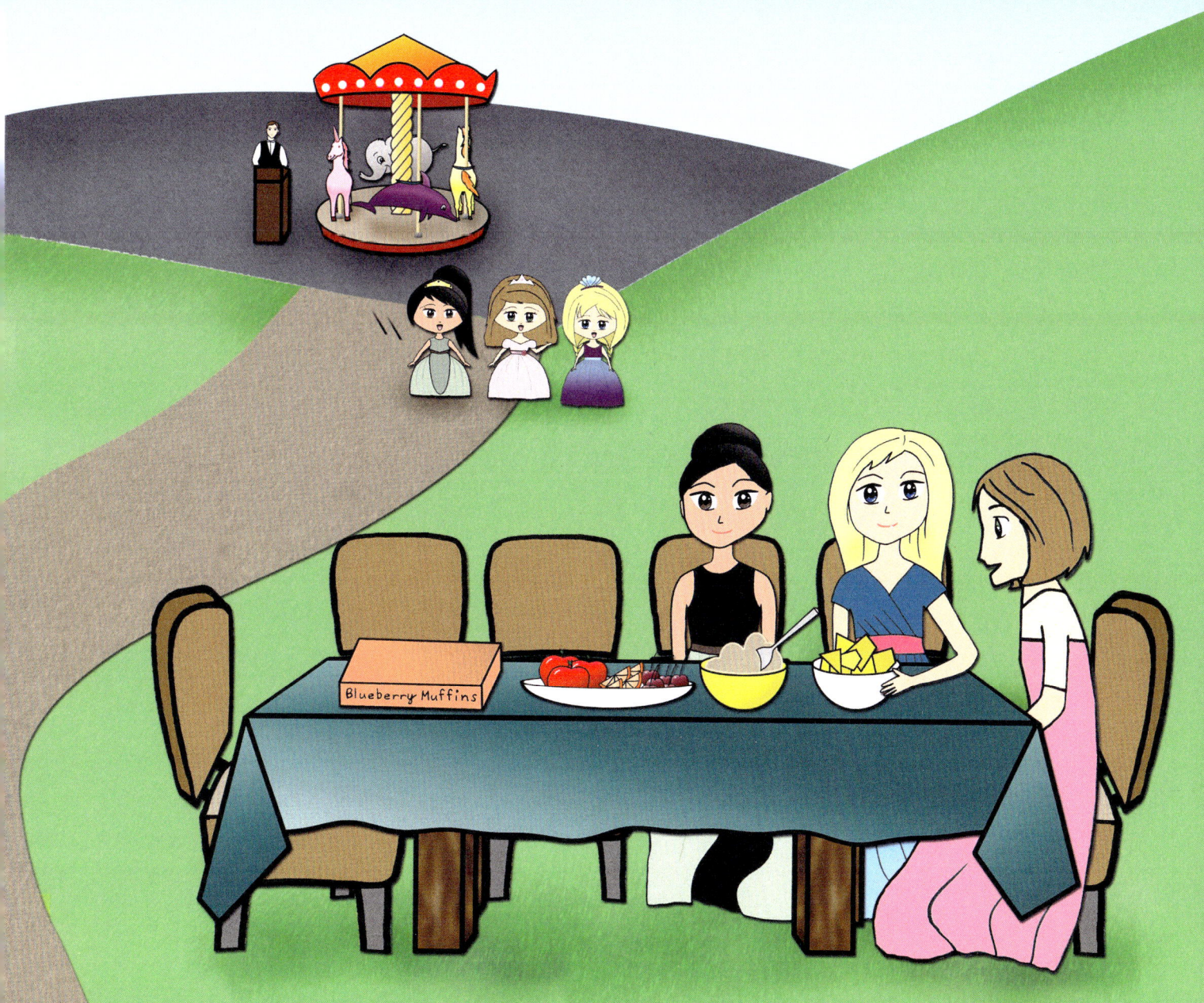

After a few more times around the carousel, the girls got off, looked at each other, and declared in unison, "We're starving!" They headed towards their mommies sitting at the picnic table.

After the children wiped their hands clean, Lexi's mommy took out a box of muffins that she bought from the bakery.

"Who would like a muffin?" she asked.

"Ooh! May I have one?" asked Lexi.

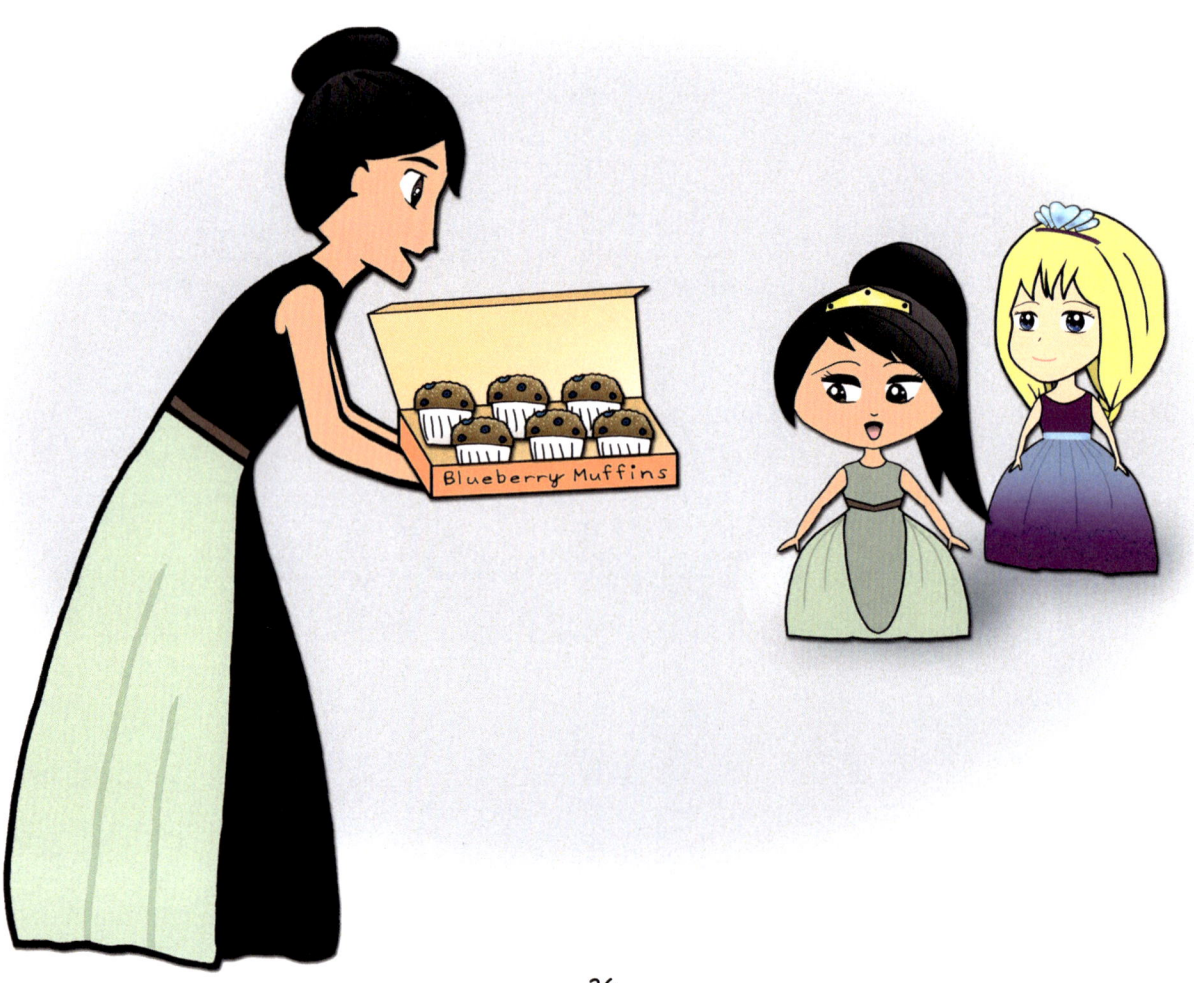

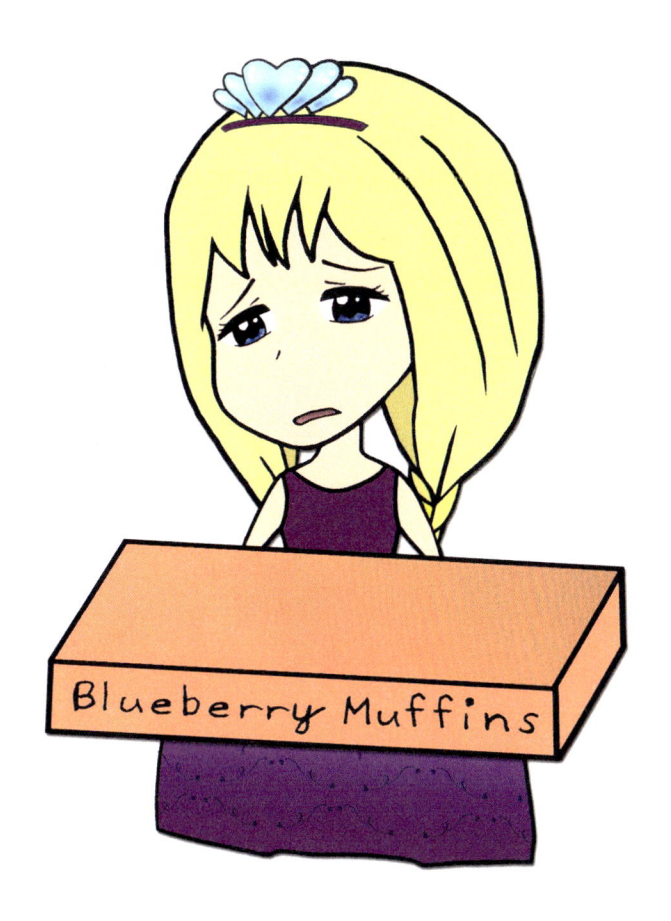

Isabella looked all over the box, but she did not see a list of ingredients. She could almost taste the blueberries and sugar crunch topping, yet she remembered her food allergies. An allergic reaction was definitely not something she wanted to go through again. She lowered her head and gazed at the ground.

"No, thank you," she replied softly.

Confused, Lexi's mommy asked her why.

Isabella hesitated, unsure of what to say, then muttered, "Well... I really want to try a muffin, but I have food allergies... and I have to be extra careful when ingredients aren't listed."

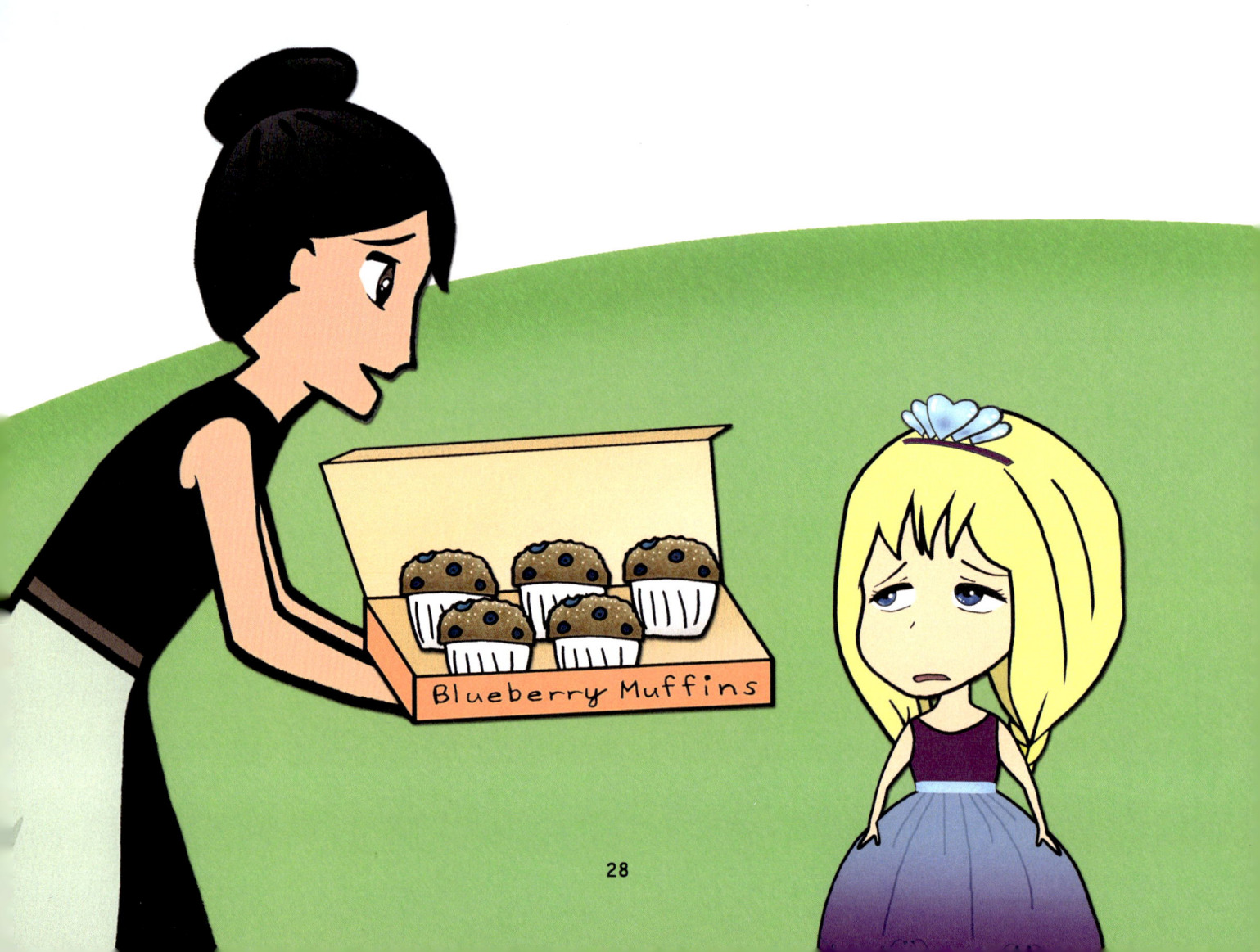

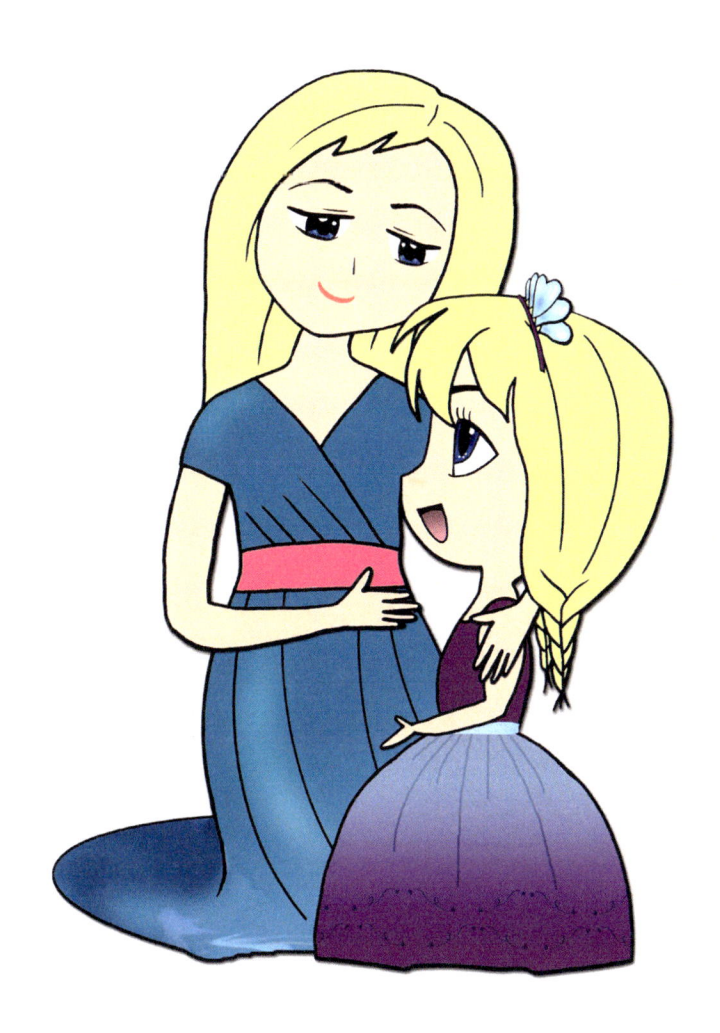

Isabella's mommy put her arm around her.

"I'm proud of you for telling our new friends about your food allergy. Friends care and help keep you safe," she said.

30

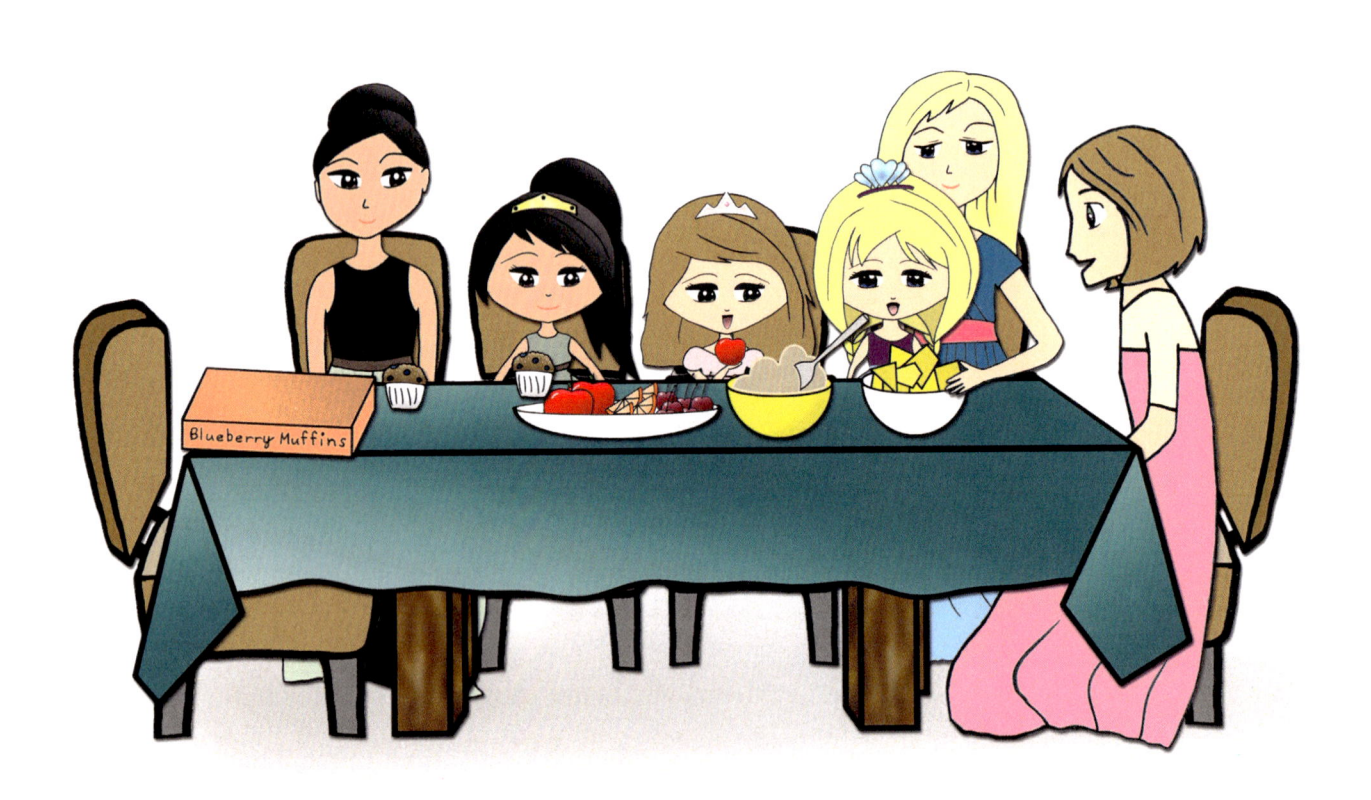

At the table, Isabella reached for the

_____.
[fill in safe snacks here]

"Thank you Mommy for preparing something safe I can eat," said Isabella.

With a loving squeeze, her mommy replied, "I'm always here to keep you safe."

THE END

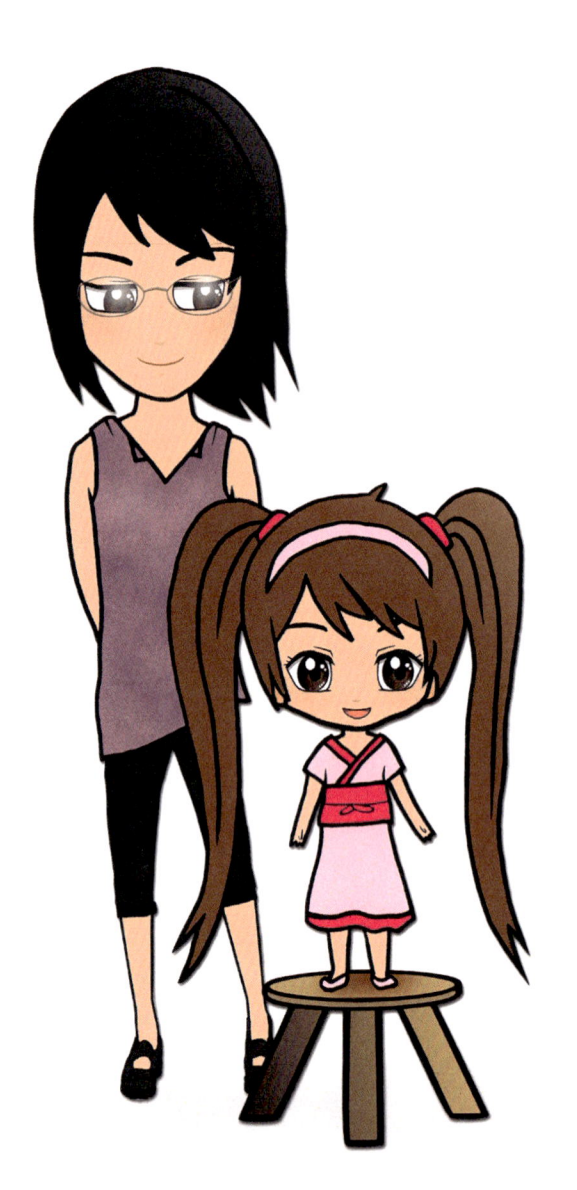

About the Authors

Jennifer Chung was motivated to create this book when she could not find one that targeted her two children's specific food allergies. Despite a love of art, she majored in Computer Science. She remembers receiving strange looks while walking into programming classes with her oversized drawing pad and pastel-smeared jeans. Working on this book with Keira has been the best mother-daughter project ever!

Keira Chung is 10 years old and lives in the USA. She loves gymnastics, violin, and art.

www.AllergicPrincess.com

Made in the USA
Middletown, DE
09 August 2018